From Your Doctor to You

WHAT EVERY TEENAGE GIRL SHOULD KNOW ABOUT HER BODY, SEX, STDS, AND CONTRACEPTION

FATU FORNA, MD, MPH, FACOG

ISBN: 149932393X
ISBN 13: 9781499323931

For my patients
and
For my children: Suma, Sinkarie, Satu, and Shekou

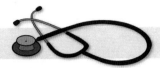

Table of Contents

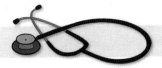

From Your Doctor to You

I wrote this book for my patients and for my children, so that they can have the information they need as they enter their teenage years. I am an Obstetrician and Gynecologist (OB/GYN), but I am also a mother, of three daughters and a son. Every teenage girl that I care for reminds me in some way of my own daughters.

At least once a month in my clinic I see a girl infected with the herpes virus who thinks the sores on her "bottom" are from scratching herself too hard; a sixteen-year-old brought in by her mother with abdominal pain who finds out she is five months pregnant; a college student who has chlamydia picked up on routine screening; or a young woman who cannot get pregnant and finds out that her tubes are blocked, probably from a sexually transmitted disease (STD) she had as a teenager.

Many of my teenage patients have not had a frank discussion with their parents about their bodies, or about sex, STDs, or contraception. Indeed, some of my adult patients cannot point out their vulva, their labia, or their urethra. My parents never said a single word to me about sex, STDs, or contraception, and I have realized that even today many parents never discuss these issues with their children. Many young people do not have access to this information at school either, as most schools do not have comprehensive reproductive health education that includes accurate and complete information about STDs and contraception. It breaks my heart each time I see a teenage patient with a preventable STD or an unintended pregnancy.

I wrote this book because I believe we can do a better job of starting discussions with our teenagers early, before they start thinking about having sex, so that they have the information they need to better protect themselves. This book is an extension of the discussions that I have with my teenage patients. It is from me to you: It is what I—your doctor, want you—my patient, to know. It contains medical advice given in an unbiased way, to encourage teenagers and their parents to start or continue discussions about their bodies, and about sex, STDs, and contraception.

To Parents

My goal in writing this book is to give girls the tools that will help them start taking control of their reproductive lives.

The book includes graphic images with real-life pictures of normal genital anatomy, and of genitals with STDs. I believe that teenage girls need to learn from real-life pictures so that they can understand their bodies. They need to see pictures, not just illustrations, of STDs so that they understand the gravity of these infections, the dangers and consequences of having sex too early, and of having unprotected sex. I believe that this will give them the information they need to be able to protect themselves from STDs and unintended pregnancies.

You might be hesitant and think that your teenage daughter is too young to talk about reproductive health, or to start learning about sex, STDs, and contraception. I want to assure you that it is indeed time to talk about these things, as your daughter probably has questions. If she cannot talk about this with you or with a doctor, she will talk about it with friends who might give her incorrect information.

You need to be prepared to have these discussions with your daughters, as most young people start having sex as teenagers. In the United States, 30 percent of teenagers have had sex by age sixteen. On average, most young people have sex for the first time at age seventeen.

Parents, let your daughter read this book, and use it to start a discussion with her so that you can guide her in making what you both think are the best reproductive health decisions.

To Teenage Girls

I hope that this book will help you to better understand your changing body, as you grow into adulthood. I hope that it helps to answer questions you might have about your body, sex, STDs, contraception, and about what to expect during your gynecological visits. I hope that it will help and encourage you to start or continue a conversation with your parents about when the optimal time might be for you to start thinking about having sex, and about how you can protect yourself from STDs and from unintended pregnancy.

Use the information in this book to start making decisions about your reproductive future. Think about when you might be ready to have sex. Do you plan to wait until you are married to have sex? Do you plan to wait until you are in college? Do you plan to wait until you are an adult? Are you planning to have sex soon? Are you already having sex?

If you are planning to or are already having sex, encourage your parents to take you to see your doctor. Make a decision now to decrease your risk of STDs by always using a condom when you have sex, and by limiting the number of sexual partners that you have over the course of your life. Consider using another reliable contraceptive method in addition to condoms to prevent an unintended pregnancy.

Start thinking of these issues now, so that you have a plan to guide your actions. Finally, partner with your parents and with your doctor to make decisions that will help you to have a healthy and safe reproductive life.

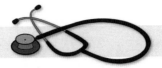

Chapter 1: Your Body

Your body is changing! I know you have noticed some of these changes. Soon you will enter **puberty**. Puberty is the stage of your body's sexual development.

What can you expect?

You will get taller and will develop breasts. You will start having your monthly **period** or menstrual cycle. You will start growing hair under your arms and in your pubic area—that area low on your abdomen. You may have acne.

Hormones cause these changes.

Hormones are the body's signals. These signals tell your body to begin to change. In just a few years, your body will change to look like that of an adult. The changes caused by hormones prepare your body for adult things, like having **sex** and having babies.

Genital Organs

If you know about your body, you can better understand all of these changes. Let's learn about your genital organs.

Your **genitals** are the parts of your body that show if you are a male or female, the sexual organs. Your **vulva** is part of the external female genital organs (**Figure 1**).

The vulva has many parts:

- The fatty area above the pubic bone is the **mons pubis**. That is where you first see hair growing.

- The **labia majora** are the large outside areas that look like lips.

- The **labia minora** are the smaller lips that are inside the labia majora.

- The **clitoris** or glans clitoris is a rod-like structure. It is above the labia minora. The clitoris is covered by a piece of tissue called the hood.

There are two openings in the external genital organs:

- Right below the clitoris is a small opening called the **urethra**. This opening is where urine passes from your body.

- The second opening is called the **vagina**. It is right below the urethra.

The vagina is an important opening to know about. Through the vagina, **sperm** enters the body. Sperm is the male version of the female egg. When a man and woman have sex, the male penis is put inside the vagina. Sperm are released from the male into the female body in this way. When the sperm meets an egg in the female body, a baby can be created. When a baby is born, it comes out through the vagina.

The vagina is also the opening where blood comes out during your period. We will talk more about periods later.

Another opening in the area below the genitals is called the **anus**. The anus is where bowel movements come out of the body. The name of the area between the vagina and the anus is the **perineum**.

The opening of the vagina has a partial covering called the **hymen**. The hymen doesn't completely cover the vagina. It forms a small circle around the vagina and has a hole in the middle. The hymen is very fragile. It will be stretched as you grow and can have small tears. These tears can happen with vigorous exercise, during sex, or when anything is put in the vagina. A tampon used during your period can cause stretching or a small tear. Stretching and small tears are expected to happen. A stretched or broken hymen does not mean that a person has already had sex.

You have learned about the vulva and its parts. Now, let's look inside.

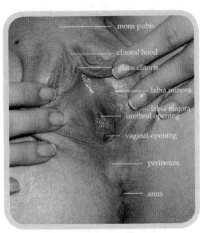

Figure 1: External Female Genital Organs

Internal Pelvic Organs

The vagina is a muscular tube. At the inside end of the vagina is the **cervix (Figure 2).**

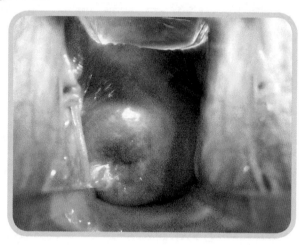

Figure 2: Normal Cervix

The cervix has a small opening in it, and this opening leads to the **uterus**. Look at the picture of the internal female pelvic organs—the inside picture of a woman's body (**Figure 3**). Your internal pelvic organs are located in your pelvis, which is the area in your abdomen between your pelvic or hip bones. The uterus is one of these organs. The uterus is where a baby grows when you become pregnant.

Attached to the top of the uterus are the **fallopian tubes**. These two little tubes are the pathways to the **ovaries**. The ovaries are the part of the body that produces and releases an egg each month after puberty starts. This process of releasing an egg is called **ovulation**. An egg can only grow into a baby if the egg meets a sperm. We call this **fertilization**, and it can happen when a woman has sex. The egg and sperm meet in the fallopian tube and form an **embryo** (tiny baby). This embryo then travels to the uterus where it grows and becomes bigger during a pregnancy.

The ovaries are also important because they produce hormones. Two of the hormones that come from the ovaries are estrogen and progesterone. These two hormones signal your body to change and cause you to grow into a woman. Your breasts will grow and you will start your period because of these hormones.

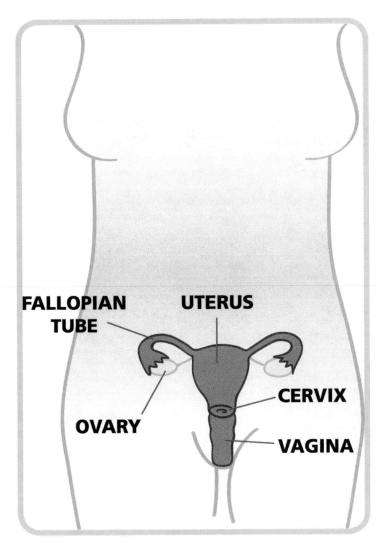

Figure 3: Internal Female Pelvic Organs

The Male Genital Organs

Let's learn about the male genital organs (**Figure 4**).

The **penis** looks like a rod and it is made of muscle. It has a single opening at the top called the urethra. This is where urine passes from the body. Sperm also comes out of this opening. At the bottom of the penis, there are two ball shaped structures called the **testicles** that are inside of a sack called the **scrotum**.

The testicles make sperm and they make male hormones. Sperm move from the testicles through a tube called the vas deferens, and mixes with fluid that comes from the **prostate** to form **semen**.

Semen is sperm mixed with fluids. Semen comes out of the urethra during sex—this is called **ejaculation.**

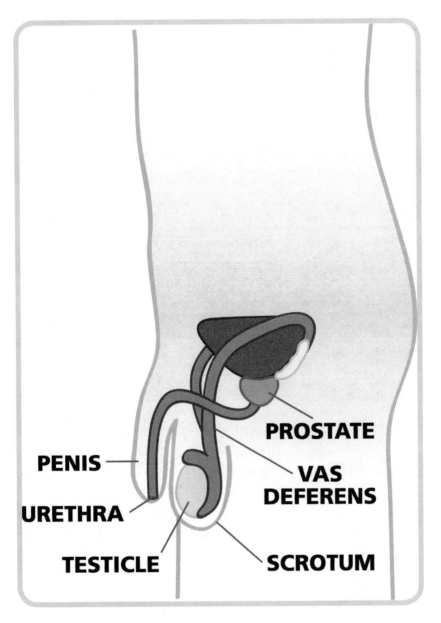

Figure 4: Male Genital Organs

Puberty

Remember, puberty is that fast-changing time when sexual development occurs. Puberty usually starts around age nine to eleven. Sometimes puberty starts later. Usually a person is finished with puberty by age fifteen to seventeen. As you go through puberty, you will notice more fat around your breasts, buttocks, thighs, and pubic area. These changes will make your shape more like an adult woman.

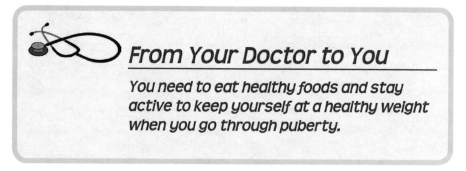

From Your Doctor to You

You need to eat healthy foods and stay active to keep yourself at a healthy weight when you go through puberty.

Here are some of the changes to expect during puberty:

- **Age 9–11: Breast development**

Breast changes are usually the first sign that puberty is coming. You will notice a lump in the middle of your breast under the **areola**. The areola is the dark area around your nipple. The lump is called a breast bud and will slowly become softer and bigger. The areola gets bigger next and you may notice another lumpy place on top of the breast bud. Over time, these lumpy breasts become smooth.

- **Age 10–12: Pubic hair growth**

You will notice a little hair starting to grow in your pubic area. This usually starts a few months after you start to develop breast buds.

This hair gets thicker and spreads. Hair will grow to cover the whole vulva. You will also have some hair grow toward your navel. Hair also starts to grow under your arms. The hair will get thicker over time.

- **Age 11–12: Growth spurt**

This is the time that you will grow taller. Usually around age eleven or twelve you will experience the growth spurt that you may have seen in older sisters or friends. You are not just getting taller; all of your body is growing. The female organs are also growing. The uterus and ovaries get bigger. The muscle of the vagina gets thicker. The clitoris enlarges. All of these changes are due to the hormones of puberty.

- **Age 12–14: Start of the menstrual cycle, or period**

About two years after you start puberty you will have your first period. Most girls get their period about age twelve. Some girls can start their period earlier or later. It is normal to start your period anytime from age eight to age sixteen.

So what is a period? You probably know about the bleeding that happens. But let's talk about what causes this bleeding.

A period is part of the menstrual cycle. The cycle starts as an egg begins to grow in your ovary. When this egg finishes growing, it is mature and is let go by the ovary. Letting go of the egg is called ovulation. Your body will produce an egg almost every month.

While the egg is growing and maturing, other changes happen. The uterus also changes during the menstrual cycle. The lining or inside of the uterus thickens with a little extra tissue. This lining of the uterus is called the **endometrium.**

When a woman is ready to have a baby, all of these changes are how the body prepares for a pregnancy. An egg is released from the ovary and begins to travel to the uterus. After having sex, sperm travel into the uterus and through the fallopian tubes. When an egg and sperm meet, this is called fertilization. At this time a pregnancy starts.

Most months no pregnancy happens and a period starts. The period is the shedding of the lining of the uterus. It is when you see the blood and a little tissue. Getting a period every month is a sign that you are not pregnant.

The first day of your period is the first day of your menstrual cycle. Most of the time you have a period every twenty-eight to thirty-two days. The bleeding time is usually three to seven days.

It takes a few years for your menstrual cycle to become regular. During your first period, the blood may be only a little brown or brownish-red spot. Sometimes you may skip a period or have longer or shorter periods. Sometimes you will see bits of tissue, which look like little blood clots. They sometimes look like bits of liver. This is all normal.

Some people feel cramps or a little pain during their period. The cramps are your uterus squeezing out the lining and the blood. Remember, the uterus is a big, strong muscle. It is normal to have some cramping. Using ibuprofen or acetaminophen may help your feel better. If you still have pain with your periods, see your doctor. There are other medicines that might help. Some women and girls take birth control pills to help their periods. You may think that birth control pills are only to prevent pregnancy. But these pills can also make your period lighter, shorter, and less painful.

Pads and Tampons

Pads (**Figure 5**) are used to collect blood and prevent it from soiling your clothes during your period. They are also called sanitary napkins.

Pads usually have a sticky adhesive patch that you can stick to your underwear. They should be wrapped up and disposed of in the trash after use. They should not be flushed, as they can clog the toilet.

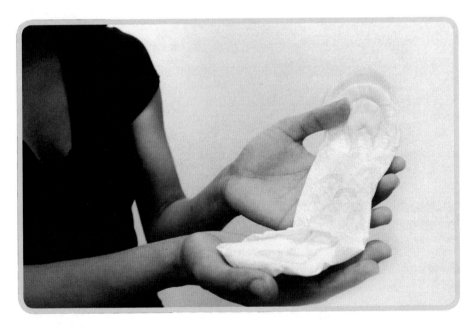

Figure 5: Pad

Some people prefer to use tampons (**Figure 6**) instead of pads, especially during swimming or exercising. You can use a tampon even if you have never had sex, but you should discuss with your mom or doctor to see if you are ready to use tampons. Tampons become easier to use the older you get because your vaginal opening gets larger. You should use the smallest possible tampon available when you first start using tampons.

Tampons usually come inside of a smooth plastic or cardboard applicator and have a string on the end. You might need an older person to help you the first time you use a tampon. You can use the tampon by following these steps:

- Insert the tampon by gently pushing the whole applicator into your vagina.

- Squeeze the plunger so that the tampon stays in your vagina while you remove the applicator.

- Stop trying to insert the tampon and get help if you have pain with the insertion.

- To remove the tampon, you just pull on the string.

The tampon wrapper and plastic applicator should be disposed of in the trash. The tampon itself can be flushed.

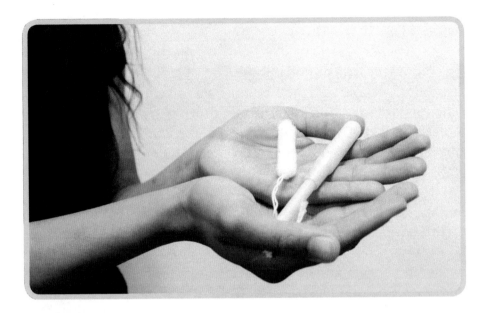

Figure 6: Tampon

It is usual to have to change your pad or tampon anywhere from 4-8 times a day. During your period, blood can have a bad smell after staying on your pad for a couple of hours. This is because bacteria grow inside the blood and cause it to break down. You should pay close attention to hygiene during your period. Take showers and clean the genital area with soap and water at least twice a day during your period.

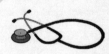 *From Your Doctor to You*

You are bleeding too much and will need to see a doctor if your pad or tampon gets filled with blood within one hour of putting it on.

Hygiene During Puberty

The hormones made during puberty can cause your skin to become oily. You may develop acne. You may also sweat more and notice a change in body odor. Bacteria can grow in sweat and cause an unpleasant odor. During and after puberty, you should take daily showers and use deodorant to help keep from getting an unpleasant body odor.

Vaginal discharge is secretions from your vagina that you might start to notice on your underwear during puberty. It is normal to have a clear or white vaginal discharge from time to time. Your vagina and cervix make secretions in response to the different hormones. Shedding the secretions as discharge naturally cleans the vagina. Because of this, you do not need any special things like scented soaps or **douches** to clean the vagina. A douche is a tube filled with liquid inserted inside the vagina to clean it. Using a douche might actually be harmful and cause infections in the vagina. Washing the outside of the vulva and the vaginal opening daily with soap and water is all that is needed to clean the genitals.

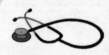 *From Your Doctor to You*

You might have an infection and will need to see your doctor if your vaginal discharge has a bad smell, if it has different colors like green or yellow, or if you have vaginal itching or abdominal pain.

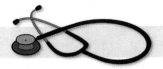

Chapter 2: Sex

Your body is changing both internally and externally. Your hormones are changing. You will notice that your feelings and relationships are changing because of all of these changes. You might notice that you are more concerned about how you look and that you take extra time to make sure you look attractive. You might notice that you are attracted to boys and that they are attracted to you. This is a normal part of sexual development, as attraction to the opposite sex is part of the way you start forming relationships. Most people are attracted to members of the opposite sex. Some people find that they are attracted to someone of the same sex.

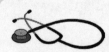 *From Your Doctor to You*

It is normal to be to be curious about sexual intercourse or sex.

It is normal to want to explore your body and to understand it better. You might notice that touching your clitoris sometimes feels good. **Masturbation** is when you stimulate yourself because it feels good. This self-exploration is a normal part of growing up. It is normal to masturbate in private, and it is also normal to not want to masturbate.

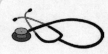

From Your Doctor to You

At some point when you start having boyfriends, you might think about what sex is and when is a good time to start having sex. Sex is something that you should consider having only when you are physically and emotionally ready to deal with what can happen when you have sex.

Sex is *any* contact between you or your genital organs, and another person or their genital organs. Many different things are considered sex. They can include:

- Vaginal sex—contact between a penis and vagina

- Oral sex—contact between the mouth and genitals

- Anal sex—contact between a penis and the anus

- Contact between the hands and genitals

- Rubbing the genitals together without actual penetration

The major biological reason for sex is to allow sperm to come into contact with the egg. This is so you can get pregnant and create a baby. Sex also brings people pleasure, so many people have sex even if they do not want to have a baby.

Having sex when you are very young and when you are not physically or emotionally ready can cause many problems. You can have emotional problems, an unintended pregnancy (getting pregnant when you are not ready to get pregnant), or sexually transmitted diseases (STDs). You should not engage in sex until you are physically and emotionally able to deal with what can happen when you have sex. Because of this, a lot of people choose to wait to have sex until they are adults. Some people choose to wait to have sex until they are married, or until they are ready to have children.

You might discuss sex, and when to have sex, with your friends. You should not let pressure from friends, or anyone else, determine when it is best for you to have sex for the first time. That is a decision that only you can make with guidance from your parents. You should discuss the best time to start having sex with your parents, an adult you trust, or your doctor. These people can guide you as you start to develop your plans for physical intimacy in your relationships.

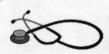 *From Your Doctor to You*

Using alcohol or drugs can impair your ability to make decisions about having sex and about protecting yourself from sexually transmitted diseases and unintended pregnancy.

Being forced into having sex is called **rape**. You can be raped by a stranger, a boyfriend, a friend, or even a family member. You should talk with your parent or another trusted adult, or call 911 for emergency services, if you have been raped. If you have been raped, you will need to be treated by a doctor as soon as possible, to help keep you from getting pregnant or getting STDs.

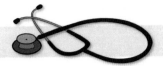

Chapter 3: Sexually Transmitted Diseases

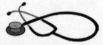

From Your Doctor to You

STDs are one of the main reasons why you should delay having sex for as long as possible!

Let's talk about a scary subject—sexually transmitted diseases (STDs). As a doctor, I want you to feel scared about STDs! According to the Centers for Disease Control and Prevention, twenty million people get an STD every year. Most of these are young people between the ages of fifteen and twenty-four. Both men and women get STDs. Women are the ones that usually have serious problems from STDs. Some of these problems can last a long time.

STDs can cause an infection called **pelvic inflammatory disease,** or PID. PID makes you sick—you may have pain in your abdomen, and a fever. PID can also cause scars in your internal pelvic organs. These scars can cause pain that can last for years, called **chronic pelvic pain**.

Sometimes PID scars make it impossible to have a baby. This is called **infertility**. Other times the scars cause a pregnancy problem called **ectopic pregnancy**. An ectopic pregnancy is when the developing pregnancy is stuck in the fallopian tube, where it cannot grow. An ectopic pregnancy is serious and some people can die from it if they are not seen quickly by a doctor.

You may have heard of some of the STDs, such as chlamydia, gonorrhea, syphilis, and trichomoniasis. A person that gets one of these STDs needs to take medicine to get well. These infections have to be treated early. If they are not treated early, a person can develop some of the long-term problems like PID, chronic pelvic pain, infertility, or ectopic pregnancy.

Some STDs cannot be cured. Herpes and HIV are two of the infections that, once you get them, you will always have them. We are going to talk a lot more about these STDs.

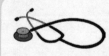 *From Your Doctor to You*

You should be aware of STDs—what they look like, what the symptoms are, and how they are spread from one person to another, so that you can better protect yourself.

How can you prevent STDs? The only sure way is to *not* have sex. The word for not having sex is **abstinence**.

If you are having sex you can get an STD.

There are some ways to help protect yourself if you are having sex. A condom can help prevent an STD. A condom must be used every time you have sex! Condoms also have to be used correctly. Later I will show you pictures about how to use a condom.

Other things you do can help. For instance, wait to have sex. You are less likely to get an STD if you wait until you are older before you first have sex. Limit the number of people you have sex with. The more people you have sex with, the greater your risk of getting an STD.

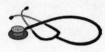 **From Your Doctor to You**

You can't trust anyone but yourself to protect your health. You are the only one who can lower your risk of getting an STD. You can lower your risk of getting an STD by:

1. *Delaying the age at which you first have sex.*

2. *Limiting the number of people you have sex with.*

3. *Using a condom each and every time you have sex.*

Let's learn about some of the more common STDs.

Chlamydia

▶ What is chlamydia?

Chlamydia is the most common STD in the United States. It is caused by bacteria. It is very common among young people. About 10 percent of sexually active female teenagers have chlamydia.

▶ How do you get chlamydia?

You can get chlamydia from any type of sex. You can get chlamydia from vaginal, oral, or anal sex. Chlamydia can be spread even if a man does not ejaculate during sex.

▶ What are the symptoms of a chlamydia infection?

Many times there are no symptoms of chlamydia. It is sometimes called the silent infection because most people have no symptoms. Chlamydia infects the cervix in women (Figure 7). Sometimes the infection will cause a vaginal discharge. It can also cause bleeding during sex or between periods. This bleeding is from the cervix being raw and infected. Some people feel pain or burning when they urinate, or empty their bladder.

Chlamydia can also cause an infection in the throat, eyes, or rectum.

Some infected men can have a discharge from the penis. Some may have a burning sensation when urinating, or pain or swelling in the genitals. Some men have no symptoms at all.

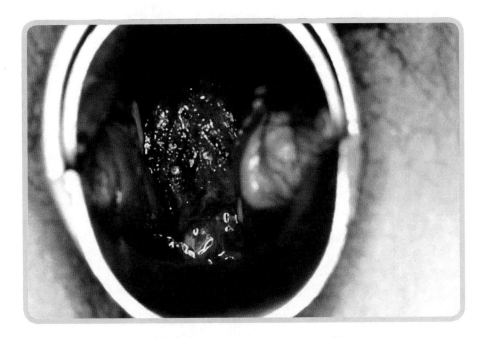

Figure 7: Cervix with bleeding from a Chlamydia Infection

▶ *What problems can chlamydia cause?*

A chlamydia infection can cause PID, infertility, ectopic pregnancy, or chronic pelvic pain. If chlamydia is not treated, a person has a higher chance of getting the HIV infection if they are exposed to HIV.

▶ *How can you test for chlamydia?*

Your doctor can test for chlamydia. Testing can be done with a urine sample, or through a swab of the vagina. This testing will pick up vaginal infections. A swab of the throat will test for infection from oral sex. A rectal swab can look for infection from anal sex. Young women who are sexually active should be tested for chlamydia once a year.

▶ How can you treat chlamydia?

Chlamydia is easily treated with antibiotics. Sexual partners also need to be treated. Both partners should not have sex for seven days after treatment, to keep from passing the infection back and forth.

▶ How can you prevent chlamydia?

Use condoms every time you have sex, or don't have sex at all.

Condoms can prevent most, but not all, chlamydia infections because infections can be transmitted through any contact with genital secretions. Contact with genital secretions can happen even if you use a condom during sex. Abstinence from sex is the only way to prevent all chlamydia infections.

Remember, you can get chlamydia during oral, anal, or vaginal sex.

Genital Warts and HPV Infections

▶ *What are genital warts?*

Genital warts (Figure 8, Figure 9) are small bumps that grow in the genital area. They are caused by a virus.

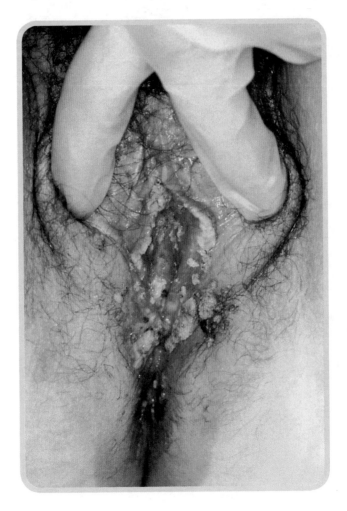

Figure 8: Vulva with Genital Warts

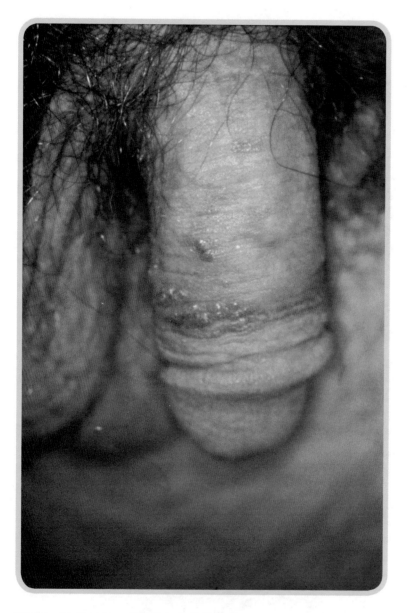

Figure 9: Penis with Genital Warts

▶ What is HPV?

HPV stands for Human Papilloma Virus. There are many different types of HPV. One type of HPV can cause genital warts. Another type can cause changes in the cervix, called **dysplasia** which can cause cancer.

HPV spread during oral sex can cause warts to grow in the mouth and throat.

HPV is the most common STD, and most sexually active people will get HPV infection at some point in their lives.

Most HPV infections don't cause any problems and they go away on their own.

▶ How do you get genital warts/HPV?

Genital warts are very infectious and are spread by skin-to-skin contact during sex. You can get genital warts or HPV from vaginal, oral, or anal sex. You can get genital warts or HPV even if you use condoms every time you have sex.

▶ What are the symptoms of genital warts/HPV?

People with genital warts will see or feel small bumps in the genital area. They are usually not painful. Women will usually have no symptoms if they have an HPV infection in the cervix.

▶ What problems can genital warts/HPV cause?

The warts can get very big and can come back even after they are treated. Untreated dysplasia caused by HPV in the cervix can lead to cancer of the cervix. HPV in the mouth and throat can cause cancer in those areas.

▶ How can you test for genital warts/HPV?

Your doctor can test for genital warts or HPV. He or she can examine the bumps and let you know if they are genital warts based on how they look. Your doctor can also do a biopsy test, by cutting off a tiny piece of the wart. Your doctor can test for HPV by taking a swab of the cervix.

▶ How can you treat genital warts/HPV?

Genital warts can be treated by a cream that you put on the warts for a couple of weeks. The doctor can also put an acid directly on the warts to burn them off. Sometimes surgery is necessary to treat the warts.

The immune system helps the body fight infections and can usually cure most HPV infections within two years. Sometimes, the immune system is unable to cure the virus and people get recurrent genital warts or dysplasia of the cervix.

▶ How can you prevent genital warts/HPV?

Use condoms every time you have sex, or don't have sex at all.

Condoms can prevent some, but not all, genital warts and HPV infections because infections can be transmitted through skin-to-skin contact. Skin-to-skin contact can happen even if you use a condom during sex. Abstinence from sex is the only way to prevent all genital warts and HPV infections.

Remember, you can get genital warts and HPV during oral, anal, or vaginal sex.

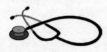

From Your Doctor to You

The HPV vaccine helps protect against getting some HPV infections. It is usually given to eleven- or twelve-year-old girls and boys, but catch-up vaccines can be given up to age twenty-six if you did not get the vaccine when you were younger.

Gonorrhea

▶ *What is gonorrhea?*

Gonorrhea is a sexually transmitted disease that is caused by bacteria.

▶ *How do you get gonorrhea?*

You can get gonorrhea from vaginal, oral, or anal sex. Gonorrhea can be spread even if a man does not ejaculate during sex.

▶ *What are the symptoms of a gonorrhea infection?*

Many times there are no symptoms of gonorrhea. Gonorrhea usually infects the cervix in women (**Figure 10**). Sometimes the infection will cause a vaginal discharge. It can also cause bleeding during sex or between periods. Some people feel pain or burning when they urinate.

Gonorrhea can also cause an infection in the throat, eyes, or rectum.

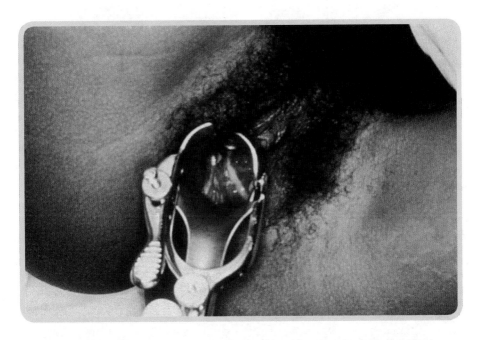

Figure 10: Cervix with discharge from a Gonorrhea Infection

Some infected men can have a discharge from the penis (**Figure 11**). Some may have a burning sensation when urinating, or pain or swelling in the genitals. Some men have no symptoms at all.

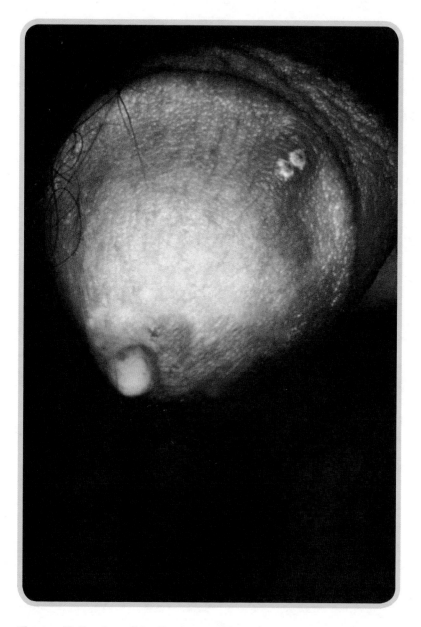

Figure 11: Penis with discharge from a Gonorrhea Infection

▶ *What problems can gonorrhea cause?*

A gonorrhea infection can cause PID, infertility, ectopic pregnancy, or chronic pelvic pain. If gonorrhea is not treated, a person has a higher chance of getting the HIV infection if they are exposed to HIV.

▶ *How can you test for gonorrhea?*

Your doctor can test for gonorrhea with a urine sample, or with a swab of the vagina. A swab of the throat will test for infection from oral sex. A rectal swab can look for infection from anal sex. Young women who are sexually active should be tested for gonorrhea once a year.

▶ *How can you treat gonorrhea?*

Gonorrhea is easily treated with antibiotics. Sexual partners also need to be treated. Both partners should not have sex for seven days after treatment to keep from passing the infection back and forth.

▶ *How can you prevent gonorrhea?*

Use condoms every time you have sex, or don't have sex at all.

Condoms can prevent most, but not all, gonorrhea infections because infections can be transmitted through any contact with genital secretions. Contact with genital secretions can happen even if you use a condom during sex. Abstinence from sex is the only way to prevent all gonorrhea infections.

Remember, you can get gonorrhea during oral, anal, or vaginal sex.

Genital Herpes

▶ *What is genital herpes?*

Genital herpes is a sexually transmitted disease. It is caused by a virus. About 20 percent of adults have the herpes infection. Herpes infection can cause sores or blisters in the genitals, but it can also cause cold sores or blisters on the lips and mouth (**Figure 12**).

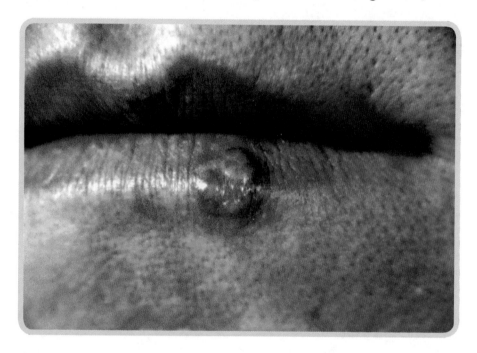

Figure 12: Lip with blisters from a Herpes Infection

▶ *How do you get genital herpes?*

You can get the herpes virus from any type of sex. You can get herpes from vaginal, oral, or anal sex. You can get herpes even if you use condoms every time you have sex, and it can be spread even if a man does not ejaculate during sex.

Most people get cold sores on their lips or mouth from kissing or close interaction with other people. These cold sores can be transmitted to the genital area during oral sex and cause genital herpes.

▶ *What are the symptoms of a genital herpes infection?*

Herpes infection can cause blisters on the external genital areas that burst and turn into painful sores or ulcers on the vulva (**Figure 13**), or on the penis **(Figure 14)**. The first outbreak is usually the worst. Herpes can cause fevers, body aches, and flu-like symptoms during the first infection. The ulcers can take 2–4 weeks to heal.

Women can also get ulcers inside their vagina and on their cervix. They can also get a vaginal discharge.

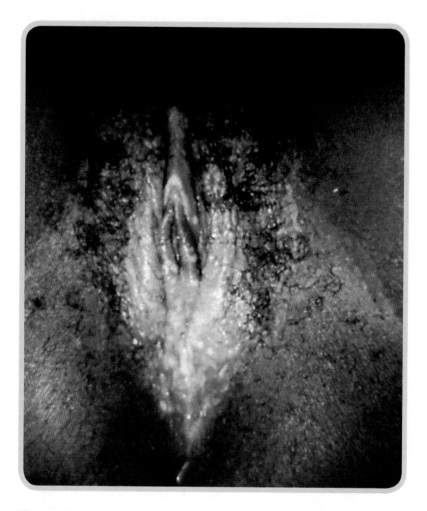

Figure 13: Vulva with ulcers from a Herpes Infection

Some people have no symptoms at all, or they get very mild symptoms. Women who have a herpes infection might think they scratched themselves, or that a yeast infection is causing their symptoms.

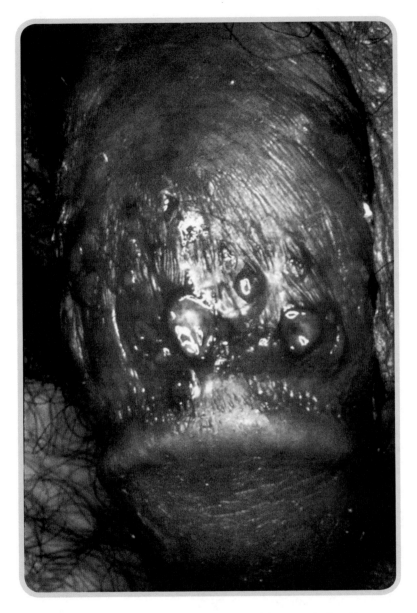

Figure 14: Penis with ulcers from a Herpes Infection

▶ What problems can genital herpes cause?

After the first infection, genital herpes can cause outbreaks from time to time. During outbreaks, you can get a cluster of blisters or ulcers that appear in the genitals every couple of weeks to every couple of years. With time, the outbreaks become less frequent. Some people stop having outbreaks after a while, but they still have the virus and can still pass it to their sexual partners.

▶ How can you test for genital herpes?

Your doctor can test for the herpes infection. Testing can be done by taking a swab of the ulcer or by doing a blood test.

▶ How can you treat genital herpes?

There are medications that can help the outbreak heal a little faster. Medications cannot totally cure the infection. People with herpes will always have the infection and it can cause blisters or ulcers from time to time.

Pregnant women can pass the virus to their babies. It is important to let your doctor know if you have a history of a herpes infection so that you can receive medication to help prevent spreading the virus to the baby.

▶ How can you prevent genital herpes?

Use condoms every time you have sex, or don't have sex at all.

Condoms can prevent some, but not all, herpes infections because infections can be transmitted through skin-to-skin contact.

Skin-to-skin contact can happen even if you use a condom during sex. Abstinence from sex is the only way to prevent all herpes infections.

Remember, you can get herpes during oral, anal, or vaginal sex.

HIV/AIDS

▶ What is HIV/AIDS?

Human Immunodeficiency Virus (HIV) is a virus that can weaken the immune system. It can make it easy for a person to get other infections. HIV is the virus that causes **Acquired Immunodeficiency Syndrome** (AIDS). AIDS is when the immune system is very weak and can no longer fight against most illnesses.

▶ How do you get HIV?

HIV can be spread by any exposure to infected blood or body fluids. You can get HIV from any type of sex. You can get HIV from vaginal, oral, or anal sex. You can also get HIV from sharing needles with someone that has the infection. Some people who inject illegal drugs in their veins share needles, which can be very dangerous.

HIV can be transmitted from a mother to her unborn child during pregnancy.

You cannot get HIV from casual contact like hugging or shaking hands.

▶ What are the symptoms of HIV?

Most people have no symptoms during the early period of HIV infection. Some people get fevers. When people develop AIDS, they can experience weight loss, skin rashes, and different infections in their body.

▶ What problems can HIV cause?

HIV can cause a person to get other infections and cancers that can cause serious illness and death.

▶ How can you test for HIV?

Your doctor can test for HIV with a blood test, or with a swab of your mouth. You can also buy an HIV test in most pharmacies and do the test yourself at home.

▶ How can you treat HIV?

There is no cure for the HIV infection, but there are different medications that can help to control the virus and help keep a person from passing the virus to other people.

▶ How can you prevent HIV/AIDS?

Use condoms every time you have sex, or don't have sex at all.

Do not share needles or syringes with anyone else.

Condoms can prevent most, but not all, HIV infections. Abstinence from sex and no contact with infected blood or bodily fluids is the only way to prevent all HIV infections.

Pregnant women who take medications for HIV infection have a very low risk of passing HIV to their babies.

Remember, you can get infected with HIV during oral, anal, or vaginal sex.

Syphilis

> ▶ *What is syphilis?*

Syphilis is a sexually transmitted disease that is caused by bacteria.

> ▶ *How do you get syphilis?*

You can get syphilis from vaginal, oral, or anal sex. You can get syphilis if you come in contact with ulcers or rashes on a person with syphilis.

The bacteria can also be spread from a mother to her unborn child during pregnancy. It can kill a developing baby.

> ▶ *What are the symptoms of syphilis?*

Syphilis can cause ulcers in the vulva (**Figure 15**) and the penis (**Figure 16**). It can also cause ulcers in the mouth. The ulcers are usually painless. They can last from three to six weeks. If a person is not treated early, syphilis can progress to a secondary stage. In the secondary stage, you can get skin rashes over the whole body, or on the palms of your hands or soles of your feet.

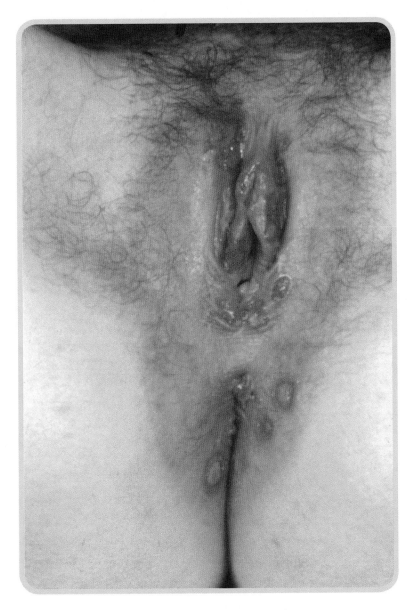

Figure 15: Vulva with ulcers from Syphilis Infection

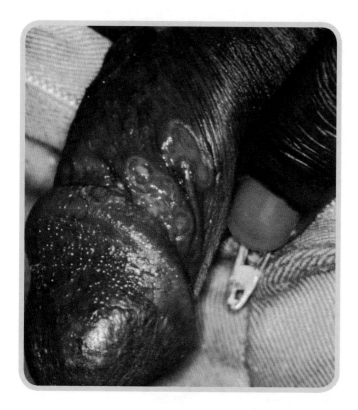

Figure 16: Penis with ulcers from Syphilis Infection

▶ *What problems can syphilis cause?*

If syphilis is not treated, it can affect the brain and cause blindness, and even death.

▶ *How can you test for syphilis?*

Your doctor can test for syphilis with a blood test.

▶ *How can you treat syphilis?*

Syphilis can be treated with antibiotics.

▶ *How can you prevent syphilis?*

Use condoms every time you have sex, or don't have sex at all.

Condoms can prevent some, but not all, syphilis infections because infections can be transmitted through skin-to-skin contact. Skin-to-skin contact can happen even if you use a condom during sex. Abstinence from sex is the only way to prevent all syphilis infections.

Remember, you can get syphilis during oral, anal, or vaginal sex.

Trichomoniasis

▶ *What is trichomoniasis?*

Trichomoniasis is a sexually transmitted disease that is very common. It is caused by a parasite called trichomonas.

▶ *How do you get trichomoniasis?*

Trichomoniasis can be spread with exposure to secretions during sex. It is usually spread during vaginal sex. It can be spread even if a man does not ejaculate during sex.

▶ *What are the symptoms of trichomoniasis?*

Women usually get the infection in their vagina or urethra. Most women don't have any symptoms. Sometimes the infection will cause a vaginal discharge and itching. It can also cause bleeding during sex or between periods. This bleeding is from the cervix being raw and infected. Some people feel pain or burning when they urinate.

Some infected men can have a discharge from the penis. Some may have a burning sensation when urinating. Most men have no symptoms at all.

▶ *What problems can trichomoniasis cause?*

The symptoms can come and go, and can sometimes last for years if not treated.

▶ *How can you test for trichomoniasis?*

Your doctor can test for trichomoniasis. Testing can be done with a swab from your vagina, or with a urine sample.

▶ *How can you treat trichomoniasis?*

Trichomoniasis is treated with antibiotics.

▶ *How can you prevent trichomoniasis?*

Use condoms every time you have sex, or don't have sex at all.

Condoms can prevent most, but not all, trichomoniasis infections because infections can be transmitted through contact with genital secretions. Contact with genital secretions can happen even if you use a condom during sex. Abstinence from sex is the only way to prevent all trichomoniasis infections.

Remember, you can get trichomoniasis during oral, anal, or vaginal sex.

Pubic Lice

▶ *What are pubic lice?*

Pubic lice are tiny insects that can infect the hair in the pubic area. They are also called crabs. Pubic lice are different from the lice that infect hair on the head.

▶ *How do you get pubic lice?*

Pubic lice are usually spread during sex or with close genital contact. Pubic lice can also be spread by sharing clothing, towels, or bedding with someone who has pubic lice. You cannot get pubic lice from using bathrooms or toilet seats.

▶ *What are the symptoms of infection with pubic lice?*

People with pubic lice will have genital itching. They might also notice lice or eggs in their genital area.

▶ *What problems can pubic lice cause?*

Pubic lice will cause itching and redness in the genital area.

▶ *How can you test for pubic lice?*

Your doctor can test for pubic lice. They can do an exam of your pubic area to confirm the presence of lice or eggs.

▶ *How can you treat pubic lice?*

Pubic lice can be treated with lotions or shampoos that are pre-scribed by your doctor. You can also buy lotions or shampoos at a pharmacy without a prescription.

▶ *How can you prevent pubic lice?*

You can prevent an infection with pubic lice by avoiding genital contact with someone who has a pubic lice infection. You should also avoid sharing clothing, towels, or bedding with someone who has an infection.

Other Common Infections That Are Not STDs

There are other infections that can cause vaginal itching and discharge that are not sexually transmitted.

Yeast normally grows in the vagina in small amounts. An overgrowth of this yeast can cause a **yeast infection**. A yeast infection can cause a clumpy white discharge. It sometimes can cause itching, redness, and swelling of the vulva and vagina. It can easily be treated with medications that you buy yourself at a pharmacy, or that are prescribed by your doctor.

Bacterial vaginosis is an overgrowth of bacteria that usually grow in the vagina. It can cause a creamy white discharge and can sometimes have a fishy odor. It is usually treated with antibiotics prescribed by your doctor.

Different things cause yeast and bacterial infections in different women. Some women get these infections if they use scented soaps or pads in their genital area, or if they wear underwear that have certain dyes that they are sensitive to.

Some women get infections if they are exposed to too much moisture in the genital area for long periods of time. This can happen if they wear tight pants that make them sweat, or if they wear wet bathing suits for too long.

Some women also get yeast infections after taking antibiotics, because antibiotics can kill the good bacteria living in the vagina. Killing good bacteria can cause overgrowth of yeast or other bacteria. Hormonal changes or medical conditions like diabetes can also cause women to get more frequent vaginal infections.

Urinary tract infections (UTIs) can occur when bacteria get into the urethra and bladder and cause an infection. A UTI can cause pain in the lower abdomen. Women can also get burning, pain, or bleeding during urination, or a feeling like they have to urinate all the time. Your doctor can test your urine to see if there is an infection. He or she can prescribe antibiotics to treat the infection.

Bacteria can get into your urethra if you wipe from your anus toward your vagina (back to front) after using the bathroom. You can spread bacteria from your bowel movements to your genital organs that way. Bacteria can also be pushed into your urethra during sex. You can prevent this by always wiping from your vagina toward your anus (front to back) after using the bathroom. You can also help prevent UTIs by urinating immediately after having sex.

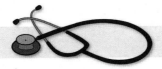

Chapter 4: Pregnancy and Contraception

Pregnancy

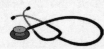

From Your Doctor to You

If you are having sex and do not want to become pregnant, you must use reliable contraception!

Pregnancy can occur anytime a woman and a man have sex. Pregnancy can occur as long as sperm comes into contact with your egg. You can therefore get pregnant even without actual penetration, if semen or sperm is deposited inside or close to your vagina.

Pregnancy can occur anytime the penis comes into direct contact with the vaginal area. This is because sperm can be present in the fluid coming from the penis before ejaculation, during ejaculation, or after ejaculation. Sperm can live for three to five days inside a woman's vagina. They can live for a few hours outside the body.

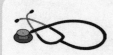

From Your Doctor to You

A pregnancy can happen if semen or sperm gets on your vulva or vagina from rubbing genitals together. A pregnancy can happen from sperm getting on your underwear. A pregnancy can also happen from sperm that is put into your vagina on a finger.

Sperm is usually put into the vagina by the penis when a man ejaculates during sex. The sperm then swim through the cervix into the uterus and fallopian tubes, where it joins with the egg. The egg and the sperm form an embryo which implants or sticks into the uterus and becomes a pregnancy. The embryo grows into a full-term baby over a nine-month period.

The first sign of a pregnancy is usually a missed period. You can get tenderness in your breasts around that same time. You may also have nausea and vomiting. You can test for pregnancy by using a urine pregnancy test that you buy at a pharmacy. Your doctor can also test for pregnancy with a urine or blood test.

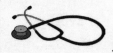

From Your Doctor to You

Talk to your parent or a trusted adult immediately if you are pregnant or if you suspect that you might be pregnant. This is so that you can get help as soon as possible.

Contraception

Contraception, or birth control, is when you use a medication or device (called a contraceptive), to help keep you from getting pregnant. There are many types of contraceptives. We will discuss some of the most common contraceptive methods.

- **Condoms** are very important because they are the only contraceptive that also protect against STDs. You should make sure you continue to use a condom to protect against STDs, even if you are using another contraceptive method to prevent pregnancy.

- **Long-acting reversible contraceptive** (LARC) methods are the most effective contraceptive choices for teenagers.

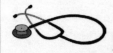

From Your Doctor to You

Long-acting reversible contraceptives (LARCs) usually work best for preventing pregnancy in all women, but work especially well for teenagers. They include the intrauterine device (Figure 17) and the contraceptive implant (Figure 18).

LARCs work well in preventing pregnancy and are much more effective than birth control pills, patches, or the ring because:

- *They last for several years.*

- *They are reversible, which means they can be removed easily and allow you to get pregnant when you want to.*

- *Once they are inserted, they don't require you to remember to use them.*

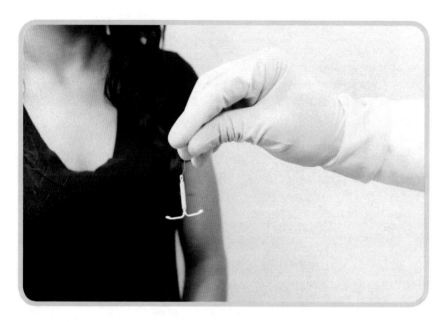

(Figure 17): Long-acting reversible contraceptive – Intrauterine Device

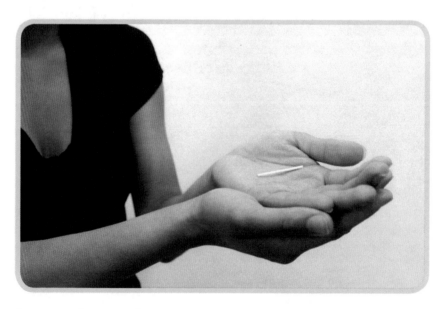

(Figure 18): Long-acting reversible contraceptive – Contraceptive Implant

Condoms

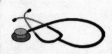

From Your Doctor to You

Other than abstinence, condoms are the best way to protect against STDs. Use a condom every single time you have sex. Other contraceptives can prevent pregnancy, but only condoms can prevent pregnancy and protect against STDs.

Condoms (**Figure 19**) are barriers used during sex to help prevent pregnancy and STDs. Condoms are usually made of latex, polyurethane, or nitrile. Condoms work by preventing the sperm from getting to the egg and creating a baby.

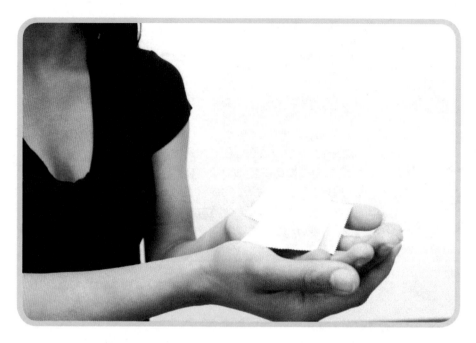

Figure 19: Male Condom

▶ *How do I use condoms?*

Male condoms are the most popular. They usually come rolled up, inside a packet. You can put on a condom by following these steps (**Figure 20**):

- Remove the condom from the packet

- Place the condom on the tip of an erect penis

- Leave a small space at the top to make space for semen, so that it does not escape from the bottom of the condom during sex

- Roll the condom down to cover the entire penis

You should only use one condom at a time—using two condoms at the same time will cause them to break or slip off easily.

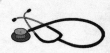 **From Your Doctor to You**

To prevent STDs and pregnancy, a condom should be used the whole time during sex. It should be put on before there is any contact between the penis and the genitals. It should be left on until the end of any sexual activity.

After sex, the condom should be wrapped in tissue and put in the trash.

Female condoms are also available, and they are inserted into the vagina before sex. The female condom is slightly more difficult to use so you might need help the first time you use it, to make sure you are using it properly.

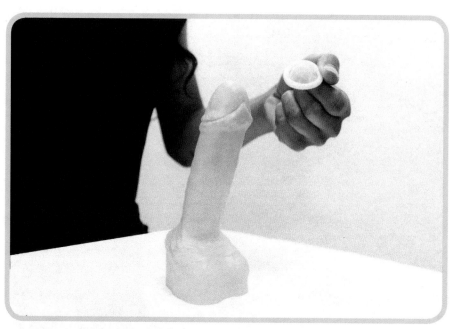

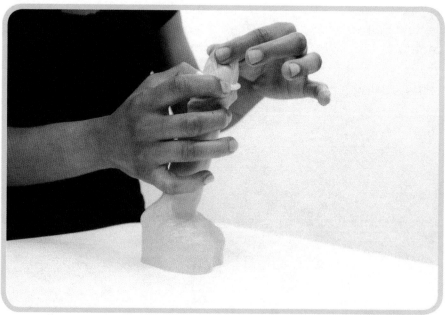

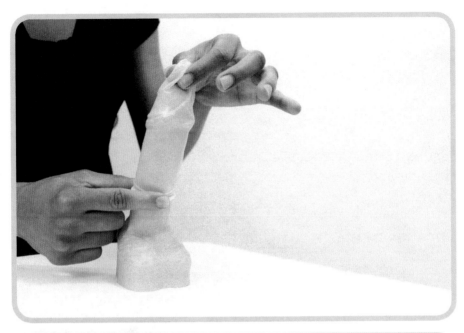

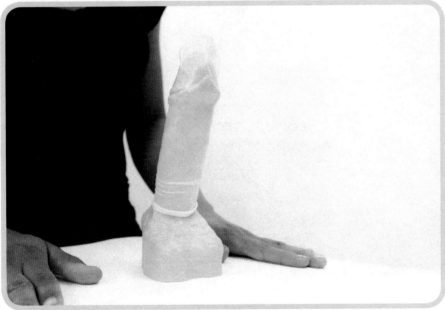

Figure 20: How To Put On A Male Condom

▶ *How long can condoms protect me?*

Condoms can only protect you when you are using them. You should use a new condom each time you have sex.

▶ *What are the benefits of using condoms?*

Condoms are very effective in preventing pregnancy when used correctly, and when used every time during sex. They help prevent against STDs.

▶ *What are risks of using condoms?*

Condoms are not effective if they are used incorrectly, or if they break or come off during sex. Doctors usually recommend that women use condoms plus another method of contraception that is more effective in protecting against pregnancy.

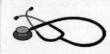

From Your Doctor to You

Dual protection is when you use condoms to protect against STDs, and use other, more effective, contraceptive method like IUDs, pills, the contraceptive implant, or the contraceptive injection, to protect against pregnancy. You should always use dual protection if you are sexually active and don't want to become pregnant.

The Birth Control Pill

The **birth control pill** (Figure 21) is commonly called "the Pill." It contains hormones. Most birth control pills contain both estrogen and progesterone, hormones that your body also produces. Another type of birth control pill has only progesterone in it. This pill is called the mini-pill.

You take birth control pills by swallowing one pill every day.

The birth control pill works by stopping ovulation. Remember, ovulation is the release of an egg that happens each month. The birth control pill is very effective if you take it every day. But if you skip days, you may ovulate and produce an egg. Skipping days will make the birth control pill ineffective and allow a pregnancy to happen.

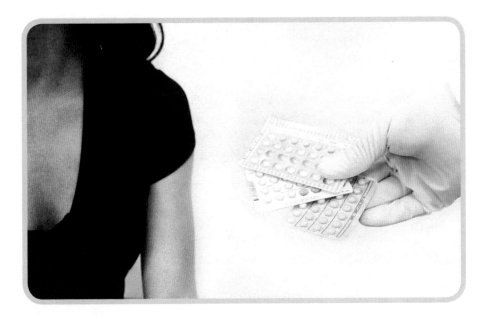

Figure 21: Birth Control Pills

▶ *How do I use birth control pills?*

Most pills come in a pack that contains twenty-eight pills. The pills are usually numbered from day one to day twenty-eight. Numbering helps you know how to take your pills. Some pills have different colors. These colors show if the pills have hormones in them. The last pills in the pack may have no hormones. They are called placebo pills.

There are different ways to start taking the birth control pill. Talk to your doctor about how to start.

Most doctors advise that you start taking your first pill during or right after your period. A Sunday start is an easy way to take your pills. For example, you would take your first pill on the Sunday after your period starts. If your period starts on a Sunday, start that day.

The first twenty-one pills in a pack have hormones in them. The last seven pills are usually the placebo pills. While you take these placebo pills, you will have your period.

Use condoms during the first month you start taking birth control pills. The pills don't start protecting against pregnancy until the second month of using them.

Pills only work if you take them! Take one pill a day, every day. Start a new pack of pills when you complete the first pack.

Sometimes you may forget to take a pill. Remember, you risk pregnancy if you miss pills. Try to take your pills around the same time every day.

▶ *What can you do if you miss a pill?*

- If you miss one pill—take two pills the next day, and then restart taking your pills again every day.

- If you miss two pills or more—take two pills the next day, and then restart taking your pills again every day.

- Don't ever take more than two pills at a time unless your doctor tells you to do so.

- Use condoms as a backup method for the rest of the month if you miss any pills in a pack.

Sometimes you may have some bleeding if you miss a pill. Your body may think you are taking the placebo pills and that it is time to have a period.

▶ *How long can birth control pills protect me from getting pregnant?*

Birth control pills only protect you while you are taking them. If you skip pills, you are at risk of getting pregnant that month. If you miss a pill, use condoms for the rest of the month. Also use condoms while you are taking antibiotics for any reason. Sometimes pills are not as effective when you are taking an antibiotic.

▶ *What are the benefits of taking birth control pills?*

Birth control pills are good protection against pregnancy. They work best for pregnancy prevention when taken every day. They also make your period regular and less painful. While taking the pills, your periods can be shorter and lighter. Some people who take the birth control pill can predict the exact day they will start having their period each month. Some women have less acne when they take the birth control pill. Pills regulate your period and make you have less acne because they can control some of the changes in your hormones.

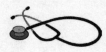

From Your Doctor to You

Your doctor can show you how to take the Pill so that you can get a period once every two to three months instead of every month, and so that you can keep from having a period during times when you don't want to have a period.

▶ Emergency Contraception

Birth control pills can also be used for emergency contraception. Emergency contraception pills are high-dose birth control pills that can be taken to help prevent pregnancy after you have unprotected sex. Emergency contraception is needed if you did not use contraception, or if you used a condom and it broke. Emergency contraception is also called "the morning after pill."

The sooner you use emergency contraception, the more likely it is to prevent a pregnancy. Emergency contraception can be used up to three days after unprotected intercourse. You can buy pills to use for emergency contraception at any pharmacy in the United States without a doctor's prescription.

▶ What are the risks of taking birth control pills?

Pills can cause some minor problems, like nausea. Some women notice nausea when they first start taking the birth control pill. It does help to eat when you take your pill. Nausea usually goes away after a few weeks.

The birth control pill does not usually cause weight gain. Pills also don't increase the risk of cancer. In fact, using the birth control pill will decrease your risk of ovarian cancer.

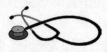

From Your Doctor to You

Any hormonal medication can cause weight gain, but the Pill does not usually cause women to put on weight.

Birth control pills can cause life-threatening complications. These complications are very rare, but are serious. These complications include blood clots in the legs or lungs, heart attacks, or strokes. Some women are at higher risk of these complications. Tell your doctor if you have severe headaches, high blood pressure, a history of heart attacks or strokes, a history of blood clots, or if you smoke. The birth control pill may not be the right contraception for you. Some women with these problems can use the the progesterone-only pill.

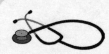

From Your Doctor to You

Stop taking the Pill and let your doctor know immediately if you start having headaches, leg pain or swelling, abdominal pain, chest pain, or shortness of breath, while taking the Pill. These are all signs of possible life-threatening complications from the Pill.

The Contraceptive Patch

The **contraceptive patch** (**Figure 22**) has the same medication that is in the birth control pill. It has the hormones estrogen and progesterone. The medication enters your body through your skin, instead of through your mouth. Some people choose the patch because they cannot remember to take a pill every day. The patch works by preventing ovulation each month.

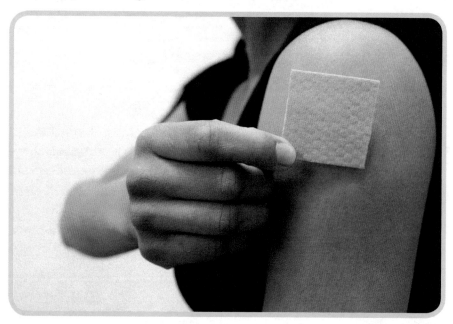

Figure 22: Contraceptive Patch

▶ *How do I use the contraceptive patch?*

Most people put the patch on their arm, abdomen, or buttock. You can put the patch anywhere on your body. It has an adhesive that makes it stick to your skin.

- You usually apply the first patch on a Sunday during or immediately after your period and leave it on for a week.

- You should switch to a new patch each Sunday for two more weeks.

- Do not put on a patch the fourth week; this is the week you will get your period.

- You can then start off with another cycle of patches the following Sunday.

▶ *How long can the contraceptive patch protect me?*

The contraceptive patch can only protect you when you are wearing it. If you forget to put on the patch when it is time to replace it, you are at risk of getting pregnant that month. You should use condoms for the rest of that month.

You should also use condoms the first month that you start using the patch, as it does not start protecting against pregnancy until the second month. You should use condoms while you are taking antibiotics for any reason. Sometimes the patch is not as effective when you are taking antibiotics.

▶ *What are the benefits of using the contraceptive patch?*

The patch provides good protection against pregnancy. The patch works best for pregnancy prevention when you keep it on the whole week, and replace it when it is time to be replaced.

The patch can make your period less painful. While using the patch, your periods can be shorter and lighter. The patch can also make your period regular. Some women have less acne when they use the patch.

▶ *What are the risks of using the contraceptive patch?*

The patch can cause some minor problems, like nausea. Some women notice nausea when they first start using the patch. Nausea usually goes away after a few weeks.

The patch does not usually cause weight gain. The patch also does not increase the risk of cancer.

However, the patch can cause life-threatening complications. These complications are very rare but are serious. These complications include blood clots in the legs or lungs, heart attacks, or strokes. Some women are at higher risk of these complications. Tell your doctor if you have severe headaches, high blood pressure, a history of heart attacks or strokes, a history of blood clots, or if you smoke. The patch may not be the right contraception for you.

The Contraceptive Ring

The **contraceptive ring (Figure 23)** is a small, flexible ring that you insert into your vagina. It has the same medication that is in the birth control pill. It contains the hormones estrogen and progesterone. The medication enters your body through your vagina instead of through your mouth. Some people choose the ring because they cannot remember to take a pill every day. The contraceptive ring works by preventing ovulation each month.

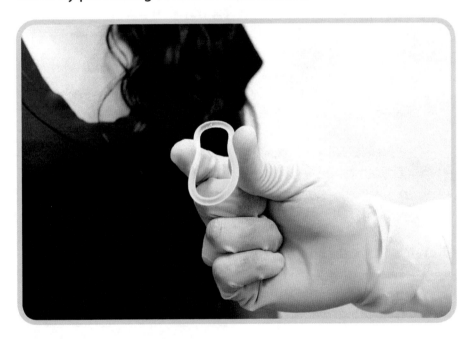

Figure 23: Contraceptive Ring

▶ *How do I use the contraceptive ring?*

You insert the ring by squeezing it in the middle and pushing it as high as possible into your vagina. You cannot push the ring "too far" into your vagina. There is no danger of it getting lost or pushed into your abdomen. The ring springs into place in your vagina and it stays in place even during sex. You will not feel the ring after it is placed in your vagina. It is alright to have sex or to use tampons while the ring is in your vagina.

- You usually insert the first ring on a Sunday during or immediately after your period.

- You should leave the ring in for three weeks.

- It is alright to re-insert the same ring immediately if it comes out by mistake during the three weeks.

- Remove the ring on the fourth Sunday after you inserted it.

- Leave the ring out this fourth week; this is the week you will get your period.

- Re-insert a new ring the following Sunday.

▶ How long can the contraceptive ring protect me?

The contraceptive ring can only protect you for the month that you are using it. If you forget to put in a new ring when it is time to replace it, you are at risk of getting pregnant that month. You should use condoms for the rest of the month.

You should also use condoms the first month that you start using the ring, as the ring does not start protecting against pregnancy until the second month. You should use condoms while you are taking antibiotics for any reason. Sometimes the ring is not as effective when you are taking antibiotics.

▶ *What are the benefits of using the contraceptive ring?*

The ring provides good protection against pregnancy. The ring works best for pregnancy prevention when you keep the ring in the whole three weeks and replace it when it is time to be replaced.

The ring can also make your period less painful. While using the ring, your periods can be shorter and lighter. The ring can also make your period regular. Some women also have less acne when they use the ring.

▶ *What are the risks of using the contraceptive ring?*

The ring can cause some minor problems, like nausea. Some women notice nausea when they first start using the ring. Nausea usually goes away after a few weeks.

The ring does not usually cause weight gain. The ring also does not increase the risk of cancer.

The ring can cause life-threatening complications. These complications are very rare but are serious. They include blood clots in the legs or lungs, heart attacks, or strokes. Some women are at higher risk of these complications. Tell your doctor if you have severe headaches, high blood pressure, a history of heart attacks or strokes, a history of blood clots, or if you smoke. The ring may not be the right contraception for you.

The Contraceptive Injection

The **contraceptive injection (Figure 24)** is an injection of the hormone progesterone. It works by preventing ovulation each month.

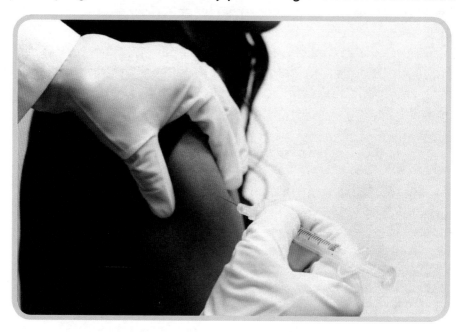

Figure 24: Contraceptive Injection

▶ *How do I use the contraceptive injection?*

The contraceptive injection is usually given by a nurse in your doctor's office. You can get the injection in your arm or buttock. You get the injection once every three months. You usually get your first injection when you are having your period, to make sure that you are not already pregnant. Having a period indicates that you are not pregnant that month.

> ▶ *How long can the contraceptive injection protect me?*

The contraceptive injection can protect you against pregnancy for three months. You have to return to the doctor's office every three months to get the injection. If you miss your next injection when it is due, you are at risk of getting pregnant and should use condoms.

> ▶ *What are the benefits of the contraceptive injection?*

One benefit of the contraceptive injection is that you don't have to take a medication every day. Another benefit is that the contraceptive injection can keep your uterus lining from growing, which can cause your periods to stop. This is normal. It is safe not to have a period when receiving the contraceptive injection. Even if you do get your period, the contraceptive injection might make it lighter and less painful.

> ▶ *What are the risks of the contraceptive injection?*

The contraceptive injection can cause irregular bleeding or spotting for the first couple of weeks to months after you first start receiving it. This usually goes away without treatment. Let your doctor know if the irregular bleeding is lasting more than a couple of months. Your doctor can prescribe birth control pills to help control the irregular bleeding.

Some women can have weight gain, depression, acne, or hair thinning with the contraceptive injection. The contraceptive injection can temporarily cause your bones to thin. Women receiving the contraceptive injection should take extra calcium to strengthen their bones. You can get extra calcium from drinking milk or taking calcium supplements.

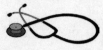

From Your Doctor to You

Most women using the contraceptive injection do not put on weight. It can, however, cause some women to put on 10–20 pounds or more. Talk with your doctor about switching to another birth control method if you notice you are gaining too much weight while receiving the contraceptive injection.

The Contraceptive Implant

The **contraceptive implant (Figure 25)** is a small plastic implant that releases progesterone into your body to provide contraception. The contraceptive implant works by preventing ovulation each month.

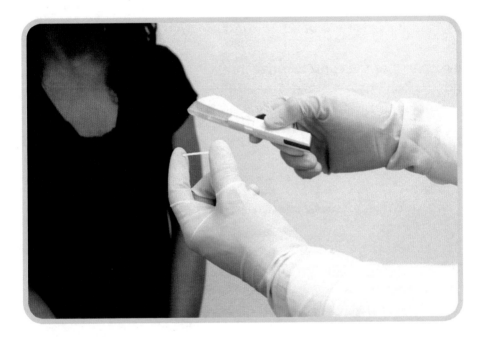

Figure 25: Contraceptive Implant

▶ *How do I use the contraceptive implant?*

The contraceptive implant is inserted under the skin of your arm by your doctor. It is not visible after it is put in. Your doctor will use a numbing medication to make sure you do not feel pain during the insertion. It usually takes less than five minutes to put the implant in your arm.

▶ How long can the contraceptive implant protect me?

The implant is a very effective method of contraception. It can last up to three years after insertion. Your doctor can easily remove it when you no longer need it. If you want, he or she can replace it with another one at the same time.

▶ What are the benefits of the contraceptive implant?

One benefit of the contraceptive implant is that it lasts three years, and you don't have to take a medication every day. The contraceptive implant is a LARC method that is especially well suited for teenagers because they do not have to remember to use it. LARCs last for several years, they are reversible, and they are very effective in preventing pregnancy.

▶ What are the risks of the contraceptive implant?

The contraceptive implant can cause unpredictable bleeding or spotting. Some women using the implant will continue to have regular periods, but some women stop having periods altogether. The contraceptive implant contains progesterone, which can cause weight gain, depression, acne, or hair thinning in some women.

The Intrauterine Device

The **intrauterine device** or IUD (**Figure 26**) is a small device that is inserted into the uterus to help prevent pregnancy. Some IUDs have the hormone progesterone. Others have no hormones at all. They work mostly by preventing the sperm from reaching the egg and causing a pregnancy.

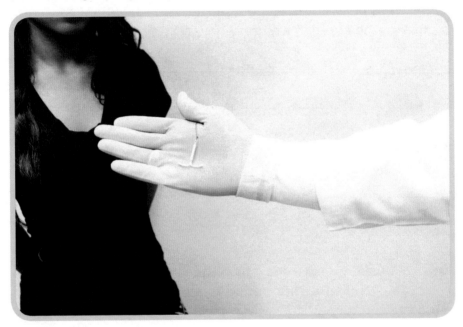

Figure 26: Intrauterine Device

▶ *How do I use the IUD?*

The IUD is usually inserted into your uterus by your doctor. You will need a speculum exam when your doctor inserts the IUD, so it can be uncomfortable to insert in someone who has never had sex. You might feel mild cramping during the insertion.

You will not notice the IUD after it is placed in your uterus. It is alright to use tampons or to have sex with the IUD in place.

Some people are worried that an IUD cannot be used in women who have never had children or in teenagers because the uterus is smaller in these women. The IUD is safe for use in women who have never had children. It is also safe for use in teenagers. There are different types of IUDs, including a smaller IUD that might cause less cramping when used in women who have never had children.

▶ *How long can the IUD protect me?*

The IUD is a very effective method of contraception and it can last up to ten years, depending on the type. You cannot remove the IUD yourself. Your doctor can remove it when you no longer need it. If you like, he or she can replace it with another IUD at the same time.

▶ *What are the benefits of the IUD?*

IUDs that use progesterone can cause your periods to be lighter. They can even cause your period to stop. It is safe not to have a period when using the IUD with progesterone. The progesterone in the IUD can keep your uterus lining from growing, which can cause your periods to stop.

A benefit of the IUD is that it lasts for a couple of years, and you don't have to take a medication every day. The IUD is a LARC method that is especially well suited for teenagers because they do not have to remember to use it. LARCs last for several years, they are reversible, and they are very effective in preventing pregnancy.

The IUD can also be used as emergency contraception if it is inserted within five days of having unprotected sex.

▶ *What are the risks of the IUD?*

You should make sure you continue to use a condom to protect against STDs. If you get an STD while you have an IUD, you can develop PID, infertility, or chronic pelvic pain.

The IUD can pierce the wall of your uterus during insertion. This happens very rarely, though, and it usually does not cause any major health problems. The IUD will need to be removed if it happens.

The IUD can also come out on its own in a small number of women. This usually happens in the first year that it is inserted.

A very small number of women can get a pelvic infection after the IUD is inserted.

You should let your doctor know if you have pelvic pain, fever, or foul smelling vaginal discharge after the IUD is inserted. This is so they can check to make sure you are not having any problems with the IUD.

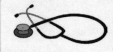 **From Your Doctor to You**

IUDs are a safe and effective contraceptive method that can be used in teenagers, and in women who have never had children.

Other Contraceptive Options

There are still other contraceptive options, such as spermicides, the cervical cup, or the diaphragm. These methods are not as effective as the others. They usually require you to use them with another method of contraception to better prevent pregnancy.

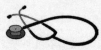 *From Your Doctor to You*

Do not use the "withdrawal method" for contraception. The withdrawal method is when you have sex without a condom, then withdraw the penis before ejaculation. You can get pregnant and get STDs with this method. This is because sperm can be present on the penis before ejaculation and cause a pregnancy. You can also get STDs, because your vulva and vagina have unprotected contact with the penis.

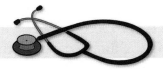

Chapter 5: Your First Gynecological Visit

The American Congress of Obstetricians and Gynecologists recommends that girls should have their first gynecological visit between ages thirteen to fifteen. This visit is usually done with a gynecologist. It can also be done with another primary care doctor or provider. Most girls will not get a pelvic or breast exam during this initial visit. The first gynecological visit is usually a counseling visit. It is usually the time when you get to meet and establish a relationship with your doctor. During this visit, your doctor will answer questions you might have about your body. You will talk about immunizations, STDs, sex, and contraception. Your doctor will usually not do an exam if you are not sexually active.

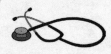 *From Your Doctor to You*

It is normal to be anxious for your first visit to the gynecologist, but you don't need to be!

Women don't have to start getting annual pelvic exams until twenty-one years of age, unless they are sexually active or they are having problems. The **Pap smear** is a screening test for cancer of the cervix. It is obtained during a pelvic exam by taking a swab of the cervix. It can be done every three years if the results are normal. Women do not need pap smears until they turn twenty-one. Breast exams are done every one to three years after a woman turns twenty-one. Girls who are sexually active need screening for STDs every year. This can be done by getting a vaginal swab, or a blood or urine test during your gynecological visit.

Depending on your history, your doctor might have to do an external-only genital exam to look for problems. If you are having any complaints like abnormal periods, pelvic pain, or a vaginal discharge, your doctor might have to do an internal exam.

During an internal exam, you will take off your underwear. You will lie down on an exam table that has stirrups that you put your feet on. Your doctor will use a metal or plastic device called a speculum to put into your vagina to look for any abnormalities. Your doctor may take swabs of your vagina and cervix. Your doctor will also use fingers to feel inside of your vagina for any abnormalities and will press on your belly to feel your uterus and ovaries. The exam is uncomfortable for some women and it can feel weird, but it is usually not painful.

Most girls will usually come with a parent for the first gynecological visit. Your doctor likely will talk with you and your parent together. He or she will then talk to and examine you alone after your parent has left the room. This is because your doctor would like you to feel comfortable during your visit. They want you to freely ask any questions and discuss any issues. Some people are hesitant to talk about reproductive health issues when others are present. But it is alright to have your parent in the room with you the whole time if you prefer.

Any issue that you discuss with your doctor is private and cannot be shared with anyone else without your consent. This is called patient-doctor confidentiality. Your doctor will ask you if you want any information shared or discussed with your parent. Your doctor will honor your wishes if you don't want information about a particular issue discussed with your parent.

As a minor, you can seek care for reproductive health without an adult if your parent or guardian can't or doesn't want to bring you for care. In the United States, nearly all states allow most minors to get treatment for reproductive health and contraception services without parental consent.

It is important for you to develop an ongoing relationship with your gynecologist so that you can get the right education and counseling about reproductive health and contraception. You should see your gynecologist once a year or as needed so that he or she can provide complete reproductive health services for you. Your gynecologist will provide care for you starting when you are a teenager and continuing during your pregnancies, if you have any, and as you get older.

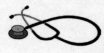

From Your Doctor to You

Talk with your parents and ask them to take you for your first gynecological visit. When you come for your visit, please be comfortable and truthful with your doctor, so he or she can provide the best care possible for you.

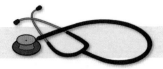

Glossary

Abstinence
Not having sex.

Acquired immunodeficiency syndrome
A condition caused by HIV infection, when the immune system is very weak and can no longer fight against most illnesses.

Anus
The opening where bowel movements come out of the body.

Areola
The dark area around the nipples.

Bacterial vaginosis
An overgrowth of bacteria in the vagina that causes a vaginal discharge.

Birth control pill
A contraceptive pill that contains hormones and prevents pregnancy.

Cervix
A structure on the inside of the vagina which has a small opening that leads to the uterus.

Chlamydia
A common sexually transmitted disease caused by bacteria.

Chronic pelvic pain
Pain in the internal pelvic organs that can come and go for a long period of time.

Clitoris
A rod-like structure in the external genitals that is above the labia minora.

Contraception
Use of a medication or device called a contraceptive, to help keep from getting pregnant.

Contraceptive implant
A device inserted under the skin that contains hormones and prevents pregnancy.

Contraceptive injection
An injection that contains hormones and prevents pregnancy.

Contraceptive patch
A patch put on the skin that contains hormones and prevents pregnancy.

Contraceptive ring
A ring inserted in the vagina that contains hormones and prevents pregnancy.

Douche
A tube filled with liquid inserted inside the vagina to clean it.

Dysplasia
Changes caused by the HPV virus that can lead to cancer.

Ectopic pregnancy
A developing pregnancy that is stuck in the fallopian tube where it
cannot grow.

Ejaculation
The process where semen comes out of the penis during sex.

Embryo
A tiny baby formed when the egg and sperm meet.

Endometrium
The lining of the uterus.

Fallopian tubes
Two tubes that take the fertilized egg from the ovaries to the uterus.

Fertilization
When an egg and a sperm meet and form a baby.

Genital herpes
A sexually transmitted disease caused by a virus that causes sores
in the genital organs.

Genital warts
A sexually transmitted disease caused by a virus, that make small
bumps grow in the genital area.

Genitals
The sexual organs that show if a person is male or female.

Gonorrhea
A sexually transmitted disease caused by bacteria.

Hormones
The body's signals.

Human Immunodeficiency Virus
A virus that can weaken the immune system.

Human Papilloma Virus (HPV)
The virus that causes genital warts or dysplasia.

Hymen
A thin membrane that partially covers the opening of the vagina.

Infertility
When it is difficult or impossible for a person to get pregnant.

Intrauterine device
A small device that is inserted into the uterus to help prevent pregnancy.

Labia majora
The large outside areas of the vulva that look like lips.

Labia minora
The smaller lips of the vulva that are inside the labia majora.

Masturbation
When someone stimulates their genitals because it feels good.

Menstrual cycle
A cycle that includes bleeding during the monthly period.

Mons pubis
The fatty area of the vulva that is above the pubic bone.

Ovaries
The organs that make the female hormones and release an egg each month after puberty starts.

Ovulation
The process of releasing an egg from the ovaries.

Pap smear
A screening test for cancer of the cervix.

Pelvic inflammatory disease
An infection in the internal pelvic organs.

Penis
A muscular rod-like part of the external male genital organs.

Perineum
The name of the area between the vagina and the anus.

Period
The shedding of the lining of the uterus that causes bleeding once a month.

Prostate
A part of the internal male genital organs that make the fluid in semen.

Puberty
The stage of sexual development.

Pubic lice
Tiny insects that can infect the hair in the pubic area.

Rape
Being forced into having sex.

Scrotum
The sac that contains the testicles.

Semen
Sperm mixed with fluids from the prostate.

Sex
Any contact between a person or their genital organs, and another person or their genital organs.

Sperm
The male version of the female egg.

Syphilis
A sexually transmitted disease caused by bacteria.

Testicles
Two ball shaped structures in the male external genitals that make sperm and the male hormones.

Trichomoniasis
A sexually transmitted disease caused by a parasite.

Urethra
A small opening where urine passes from the body.

Urinary tract infections
An infection that occurs when bacteria get into the urethra and
   bladder.

Uterus
A part of the internal pelvic organs where a baby grows during
   pregnancy.

Vagina
The opening that connects the external genital organs to the internal pelvic organs.

Vaginal discharge
Secretions from the vagina that can be normal or abnormal.

Vulva
The external female genital organs.

Yeast infection
An overgrowth of yeast in the vagina that can cause a vaginal
   infection.

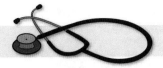

Photo Credits

Figure 1: Wikimedia. http://commons.wikimedia.org/wiki/File:Azvag.jpg

Figure 2: Wikimedia. http://commons.wikimedia.org/wiki/File:Cervix.jpg

Figures 7–16: Centers for Disease Control and Prevention, Public Health Information Library. http://phil.cdc.gov/phil/home.asp

About the Author

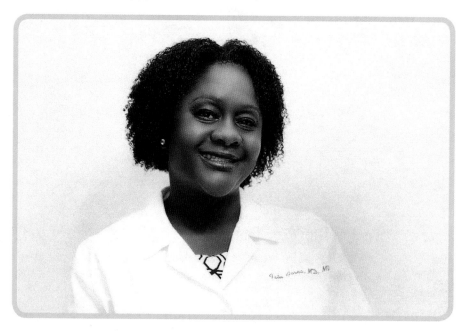

Dr. Fatu Forna received her undergraduate degree from Florida A&M University and her public health degree from the University of North Carolina at Chapel Hill School of Public Health. She received her medical degree from Duke University School of Medicine and she completed her Obstetrics and Gynecology residency at Emory University School of Medicine.

Dr. Forna served four years as a Medical Officer in the US Public Health Service at the Centers for Disease Control and Prevention (CDC). While at the CDC, she worked with HIV prevention programs in the United States and in countries around the world. Dr. Forna has authored numerous articles on STDs, maternal and child health, and HIV prevention and care. She is currently an Obstetrician and Gynecologist in practice in Atlanta, Georgia.

Dr. Forna is Co-Founder and Co-Executive Director of a nonprofit organization called The Mama-Pikin Foundation, which works to improve the health of women, children, and families in Sierra Leone, West Africa. She is married to a pediatrician, has four children, and lives in Atlanta.

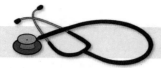

Sex, STDs, and contraception are challenging but necessary topics of discussion between parents and their daughters. This book is written by a gynecologist, and contains frank medical advice given in an easy to read, and unbiased way to encourage teenage girls and their parents to start, or continue discussions about their bodies, sex, STDs, and contraception. It is from your doctor to you, includes real life pictures, discusses what to expect during that first gynecological visit, and includes what every teenage girl should know as they grow into adulthood.